This Journal

BELONGS TO

_____

_____

Dedication

This Depression Journal Log book is dedicated to all the warriors out there who suffer from depression and want to document their findings in the process of becoming the best version of yourself.

You are my inspiration for producing books and I'm honored to be a part of keeping all of your Depression notes and records organized.

This journal notebook will help you record your details about your depression.

Thoughtfully put together with these sections to record:

Weekly Behavior Tracker, What Did I Struggle With This Week, How Did I Deal With My Depression Issues This Week, Notes, & Daily Self Esteem Page.

How to use this Book

The purpose of this book is to keep all of your Depression notes all in one place. It will help keep you organized.

This Depression Journal will allow you to accurately document every detail about your depression. It's a great way to chart your course by becoming the best version of you.

Here are examples of the prompts for you to fill in and write about your experience in this book:

1. **Weekly Behavior Tracker** - Unhealthy Habit Tracker For Substance Abuse, Self Harm, Over Spending, Over Eating, Violence, Anger & blank spaces to add your own. Checkboxes for each day.

2. **What Did I Struggle With This Week** - Track your struggles for the week.

3. **How Did I Deal With My Depression & Issues This Week** - Record how you handled your depression, what worked, what didn't, etc.

4. **Notes** - Blank lined to write thoughts of gratitude, find a way to cope with stress, ways to clear your mind, things you love doing, how you feel, happiness goals, symptoms, healthy choices, questions for the doctor, how to better control & manage your anger, etc.

5. **Daily Self Esteem Page** - Prompts include: Something I did well today, I had fun today when, I felt proud when, I had a positive experience with, Something good I did for someone else, Today was interesting because, Today's positive emotions, and Today's negative emotions.

Enjoy!

Weekly
BEHAVIOR TRACKER

Unhealthy Habits

	M	T	W	T	F	S	S
Substance Abuse							
Self-harm							
Over spending							
Over eating							
Lying							
Stealing/Cheating							
Violence/Anger							

What did I struggle most with this week?

How did I deal with my depression and issues this week?

Notes

_____
_____
_____
_____
_____
_____
_____
_____
_____
_____
_____
_____
_____
_____

Daily

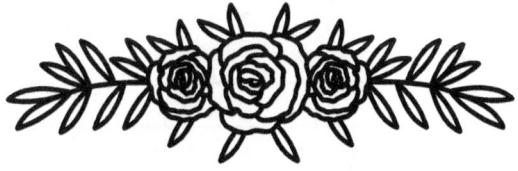

Date
_____

SELF-ESTEEM

Something I did well today

_____

_____

I had fun today when...

_____

_____

I felt proud when...

_____

_____

I had a positive experience with...

_____

_____

Something good I did for someone else

_____

_____

I felt good about myself when...

_____

_____

Today was interesting because...

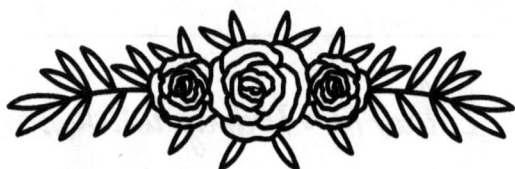

_____

_____

_____

_____

Today's Positive Emotions

Today's Negative Emotions

_____

_____

Weekly
BEHAVIOR TRACKER

Unhealthy Habits

	M	T	W	T	F	S	S
Substance Abuse							
Self-harm							
Over spending							
Over eating							
Lying							
Stealing/Cheating							
Violence/Anger							

What did I struggle most with this week?

How did I deal with my depression and issues this week?

Notes
_____
_____
_____
_____
_____
_____
_____
_____
_____
_____
_____
_____
_____
_____
_____
_____

Daily

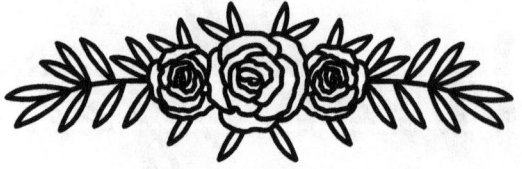

Date
____

SELF-ESTEEM

Something I did well today

_____

_____

I had fun today when...

_____

_____

I felt proud when...

_____

_____

I had a positive experience with...

_____

_____

Something good I did for someone else

_____

_____

I felt good about myself when...

_____

_____

Today was interesting because...

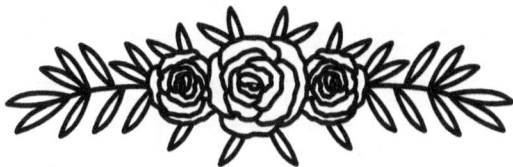

_____

_____

_____

_____

Today's Positive Emotions

Today's Negative Emotions

_____

_____

Weekly
BEHAVIOR TRACKER

Unhealthy Habits

	M	T	W	T	F	S	S
Substance Abuse							
Self-harm							
Over spending							
Over eating							
Lying							
Stealing/Cheating							
Violence/Anger							

What did I struggle most with this week?

How did I deal with my depression and issues this week?

Notes

Daily

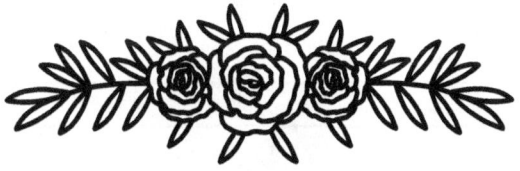

Date
_____

SELF-ESTEEM

Something I did well today

_____

_____

I had fun today when...

_____

_____

I felt proud when...

_____

_____

I had a positive experience with...

_____

_____

Something good I did for someone else

_____

_____

I felt good about myself when...

_____

_____

Today was interesting because...

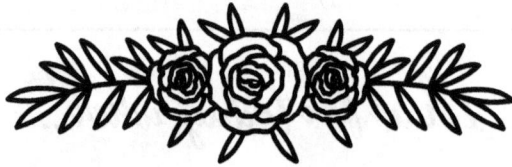

_____

_____

_____

_____

Today's Positive Emotions

Today's Negative Emotions

_____

_____

Weekly
BEHAVIOR TRACKER

Unhealthy Habits

	M	T	W	T	F	S	S
Substance Abuse							
Self-harm							
Over spending							
Over eating							
Lying							
Stealing/Cheating							
Violence/Anger							

What did I struggle most with this week?

How did I deal with my depression and issues this week?

Notes
_____
_____
_____
_____
_____
_____
_____
_____
_____
_____
_____
_____
_____
_____
_____

Daily

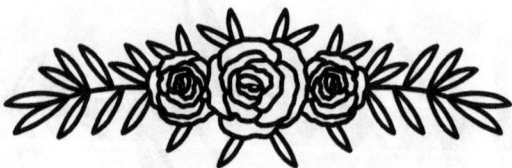

Date
_____

SELF-ESTEEM

Something I did well today

_____
_____

I had fun today when...

_____
_____

I felt proud when...

_____
_____

I had a positive experience with...

_____
_____

Something good I did for someone else

_____
_____

I felt good about myself when...

_____

_____

Today was interesting because...

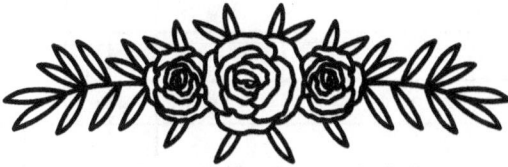

_____

_____

_____

_____

Today's Positive Emotions

Today's Negative Emotions

_____

_____

Weekly
BEHAVIOR TRACKER

Unhealthy Habits

	M	T	W	T	F	S	S
Substance Abuse							
Self-harm							
Over spending							
Over eating							
Lying							
Stealing/Cheating							
Violence/Anger							

What did I struggle most with this week?

How did I deal with my depression and issues this week?

Notes

Daily

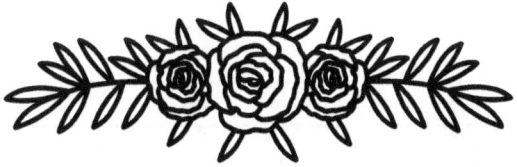

Date _____

SELF-ESTEEM

Something I did well today

_____

_____

I had fun today when...

_____

_____

I felt proud when...

_____

_____

I had a positive experience with...

_____

_____

Something good I did for someone else

_____

_____

I felt good about myself when...

_____

_____

Today was interesting because...

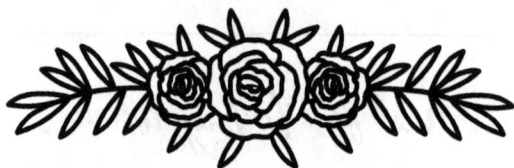

_____

_____

_____

_____

Today's Positive Emotions

Today's Negative Emotions

_____

_____

Weekly
BEHAVIOR TRACKER

Unhealthy Habits

	M	T	W	T	F	S	S
Substance Abuse							
Self-harm							
Over spending							
Over eating							
Lying							
Stealing/Cheating							
Violence/Anger							

What did I struggle most with this week?

How did I deal with my depression and issues this week?

Notes

Daily

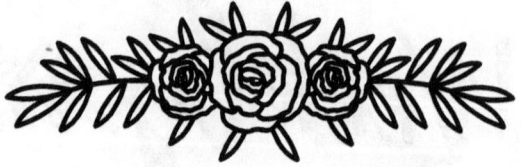

Date

____

SELF-ESTEEM

Something I did well today

_____

_____

I had fun today when...

_____

_____

I felt proud when...

_____

_____

I had a positive experience with...

_____

_____

Something good I did for someone else

_____

_____

I felt good about myself when...

_____

_____

Today was interesting because...

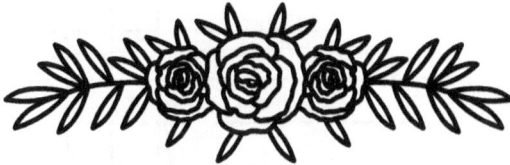

_____

_____

_____

_____

Today's Positive Emotions

Today's Negative Emotions

_____

_____

Weekly
BEHAVIOR TRACKER

Unhealthy Habits

	M	T	W	T	F	S	S
Substance Abuse							
Self-harm							
Over spending							
Over eating							
Lying							
Stealing/Cheating							
Violence/Anger							

What did I struggle most with this week?

How did I deal with my depression and issues this week?

Notes

Daily

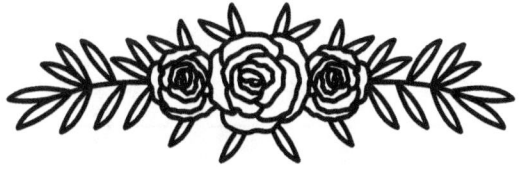

Date _____

SELF-ESTEEM

Something I did well today

_____

_____

I had fun today when...

_____

_____

I felt proud when...

_____

_____

I had a positive experience with...

_____

_____

Something good I did for someone else

_____

_____

I felt good about myself when...

_____

_____

Today was interesting because...

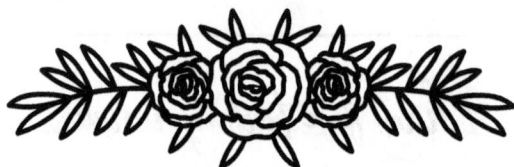

_____

_____

_____

_____

Today's Positive Emotions

Today's Negative Emotions

_____

_____

Weekly
BEHAVIOR TRACKER

Unhealthy Habits

	M	T	W	T	F	S	S
Substance Abuse							
Self-harm							
Over spending							
Over eating							
Lying							
Stealing/Cheating							
Violence/Anger							

What did I struggle most with this week?

How did I deal with my depression and issues this week?

Notes

Daily

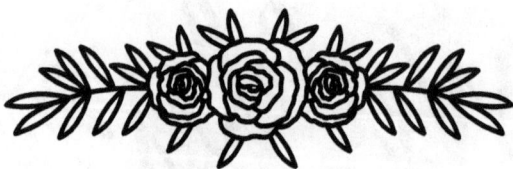

Date
____

SELF-ESTEEM

Something I did well today

_____

_____

I had fun today when...

_____

_____

I felt proud when...

_____

_____

I had a positive experience with...

_____

_____

Something good I did for someone else

_____

_____

I felt good about myself when...

_____

_____

Today was interesting because...

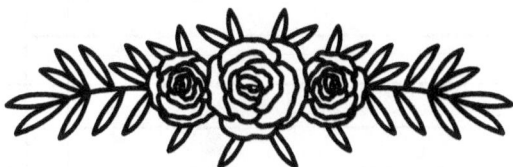

_____

_____

_____

_____

Today's Positive Emotions

Today's Negative Emotions

_____

_____

Weekly
BEHAVIOR TRACKER

Unhealthy Habits

	M	T	W	T	F	S	S
Substance Abuse							
Self-harm							
Over spending							
Over eating							
Lying							
Stealing/Cheating							
Violence/Anger							

What did I struggle most with this week?

How did I deal with my depression and issues this week?

Notes

Daily

Date
_____

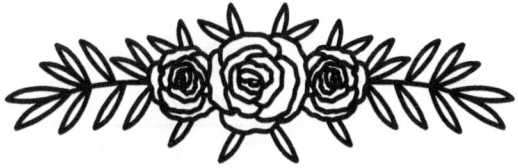

SELF-ESTEEM

Something I did well today

_____

_____

I had fun today when...

_____

_____

I felt proud when...

_____

_____

I had a positive experience with...

_____

_____

Something good I did for someone else

_____

_____

I felt good about myself when...

_____
_____

Today was interesting because...

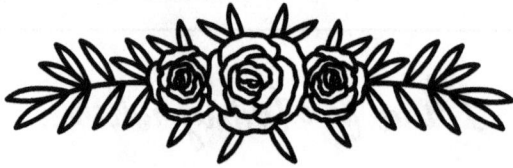

_____
_____
_____
_____

Today's Positive Emotions

Today's Negative Emotions

_____
_____

Weekly
BEHAVIOR TRACKER

Unhealthy Habits

	M	T	W	T	F	S	S
Substance Abuse							
Self-harm							
Over spending							
Over eating							
Lying							
Stealing/Cheating							
Violence/Anger							

What did I struggle most with this week?

How did I deal with my depression and issues this week?

Notes

Daily

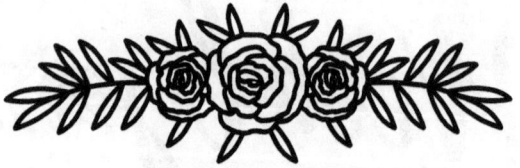

Date
_____ SELF-ESTEEM

Something I did well today

_____

_____

I had fun today when...

_____

_____

I felt proud when...

_____

_____

I had a positive experience with...

_____

_____

Something good I did for someone else

_____

_____

I felt good about myself when...

_____

_____

Today was interesting because...

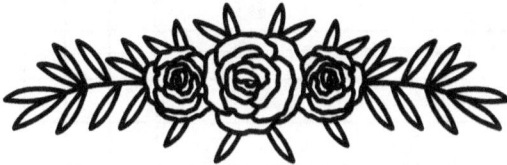

_____

_____

_____

_____

Today's Positive Emotions

Today's Negative Emotions

_____

_____

Weekly
BEHAVIOR TRACKER

Unhealthy Habits

	M	T	W	T	F	S	S
Substance Abuse							
Self-harm							
Over spending							
Over eating							
Lying							
Stealing/Cheating							
Violence/Anger							

What did I struggle most with this week?

How did I deal with my depression and issues this week?

Notes

Daily

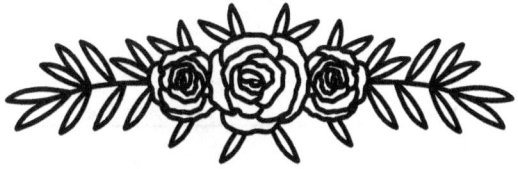

Date _____

SELF-ESTEEM

Something I did well today

_____

_____

I had fun today when...

_____

_____

I felt proud when...

_____

_____

I had a positive experience with...

_____

_____

Something good I did for someone else

_____

_____

I felt good about myself when...

_____

_____

Today was interesting because...

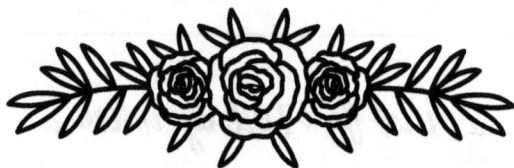

_____

_____

_____

_____

Today's Positive Emotions

Today's Negative Emotions

_____

_____

Weekly
BEHAVIOR TRACKER

Unhealthy Habits

	M	T	W	T	F	S	S
Substance Abuse							
Self-harm							
Over spending							
Over eating							
Lying							
Stealing/Cheating							
Violence/Anger							

What did I struggle most with this week?

How did I deal with my depression and issues this week?

Notes

Daily

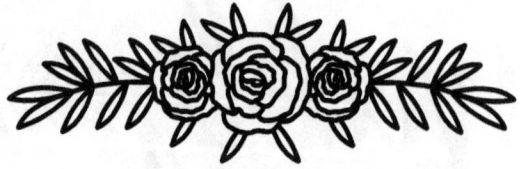

Date
____

SELF-ESTEEM

Something I did well today

_____
_____

I had fun today when...

_____
_____

I felt proud when...

_____
_____

I had a positive experience with...

_____
_____

Something good I did for someone else

_____
_____

I felt good about myself when...

_____

_____

Today was interesting because...

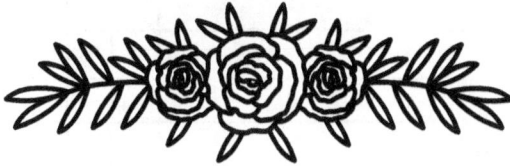

_____

_____

_____

_____

Today's Positive Emotions

Today's Negative Emotions

_____

_____

Weekly
BEHAVIOR TRACKER

Unhealthy Habits

	M	T	W	T	F	S	S
Substance Abuse							
Self-harm							
Over spending							
Over eating							
Lying							
Stealing/Cheating							
Violence/Anger							

What did I struggle most with this week?

How did I deal with my depression and issues this week?

Notes

Daily

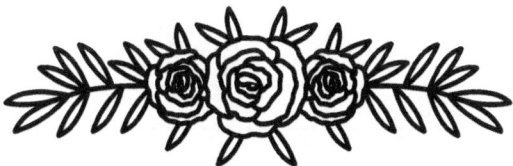

Date
_____

SELF-ESTEEM

Something I did well today

_____

_____

I had fun today when...

_____

_____

I felt proud when...

_____

_____

I had a positive experience with...

_____

_____

Something good I did for someone else

_____

_____

I felt good about myself when...

_____

_____

Today was interesting because...

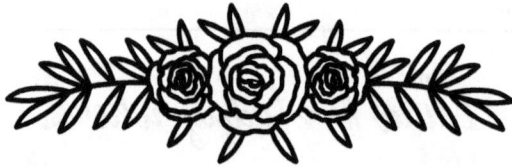

_____

_____

_____

_____

Today's Positive Emotions

Today's Negative Emotions

_____

_____

Weekly
BEHAVIOR TRACKER

Unhealthy Habits

	M	T	W	T	F	S	S
Substance Abuse							
Self-harm							
Over spending							
Over eating							
Lying							
Stealing/Cheating							
Violence/Anger							

What did I struggle most with this week?

How did I deal with my depression and issues this week?

Notes

Daily

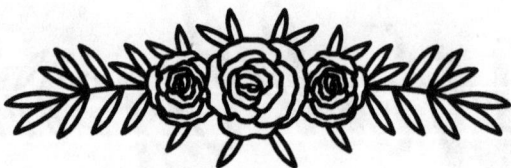

Date
____

SELF-ESTEEM

Something I did well today

_____

_____

I had fun today when...

_____

_____

I felt proud when...

_____

_____

I had a positive experience with...

_____

_____

Something good I did for someone else

_____

_____

I felt good about myself when...

_____
_____

Today was interesting because...

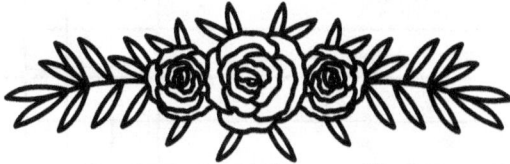

_____
_____
_____
_____

Today's Positive Emotions

Today's Negative Emotions

_____
_____

Weekly
BEHAVIOR TRACKER

Unhealthy Habits

	M	T	W	T	F	S	S
Substance Abuse							
Self-harm							
Over spending							
Over eating							
Lying							
Stealing/Cheating							
Violence/Anger							

What did I struggle most with this week?

How did I deal with my depression and issues this week?

Notes

Daily

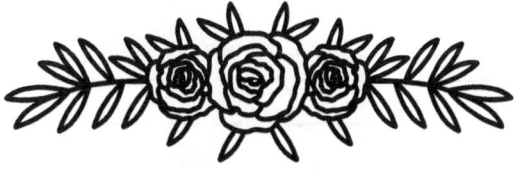

Date
_____

SELF-ESTEEM

Something I did well today

_____

_____

I had fun today when...

_____

_____

I felt proud when...

_____

_____

I had a positive experience with...

_____

_____

Something good I did for someone else

_____

_____

I felt good about myself when...

_____

_____

Today was interesting because...

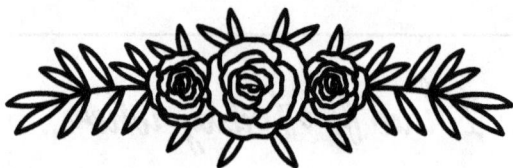

_____

_____

_____

_____

Today's Positive Emotions

Today's Negative Emotions

_____

_____

Weekly
BEHAVIOR TRACKER

Unhealthy Habits

	M	T	W	T	F	S	S
Substance Abuse							
Self-harm							
Over spending							
Over eating							
Lying							
Stealing/Cheating							
Violence/Anger							

What did I struggle most with this week?

How did I deal with my depression and issues this week?

Notes
_____
_____
_____
_____
_____
_____
_____
_____
_____
_____
_____
_____
_____
_____
_____
_____
_____

Daily

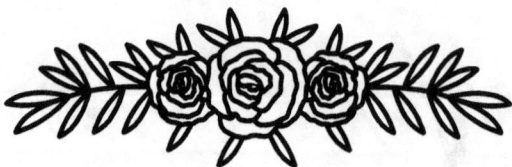

Date
____ SELF-ESTEEM

Something I did well today

_____

_____

I had fun today when...

_____

_____

I felt proud when...

_____

_____

I had a positive experience with...

_____

_____

Something good I did for someone else

_____

_____

I felt good about myself when...

_____

_____

Today was interesting because...

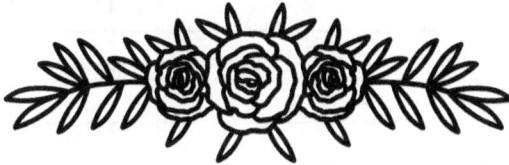

_____

_____

_____

_____

Today's Positive Emotions

Today's Negative Emotions

_____

_____

Weekly
BEHAVIOR TRACKER

Unhealthy Habits

	M	T	W	T	F	S	S
Substance Abuse							
Self-harm							
Over spending							
Over eating							
Lying							
Stealing/Cheating							
Violence/Anger							

What did I struggle most with this week?

How did I deal with my depression and issues this week?

Notes

Daily

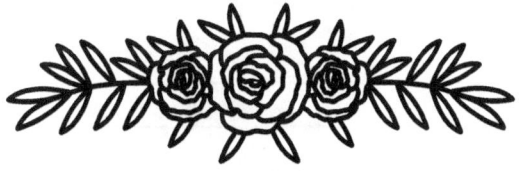

Date
_____ ## SELF-ESTEEM

Something I did well today

_____

_____

I had fun today when...

_____

_____

I felt proud when...

_____

_____

I had a positive experience with...

_____

_____

Something good I did for someone else

_____

_____

I felt good about myself when...

_____

_____

Today was interesting because...

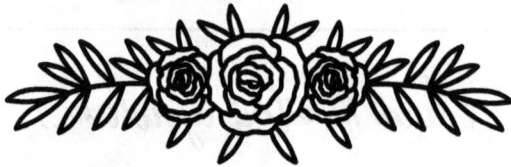

_____

_____

_____

_____

Today's Positive Emotions	Today's Negative Emotions

_____

_____

Weekly
BEHAVIOR TRACKER

Unhealthy Habits

	M	T	W	T	F	S	S
Substance Abuse							
Self-harm							
Over spending							
Over eating							
Lying							
Stealing/Cheating							
Violence/Anger							

What did I struggle most with this week?

How did I deal with my depression and issues this week?

Notes

Daily

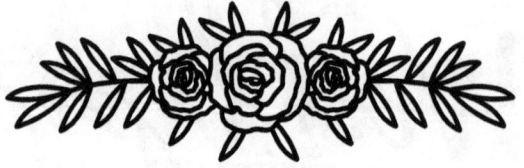

Date
____

SELF-ESTEEM

Something I did well today

_____
_____

I had fun today when...

_____
_____

I felt proud when...

_____
_____

I had a positive experience with...

_____
_____

Something good I did for someone else

_____
_____

I felt good about myself when...

_____

_____

Today was interesting because...

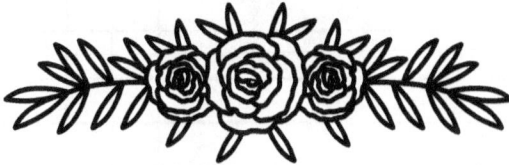

_____

_____

_____

_____

Today's Positive Emotions

Today's Negative Emotions

_____

_____

Weekly
BEHAVIOR TRACKER

Unhealthy Habits

	M	T	W	T	F	S	S
Substance Abuse							
Self-harm							
Over spending							
Over eating							
Lying							
Stealing/Cheating							
Violence/Anger							

What did I struggle most with this week?

How did I deal with my depression and issues this week?

Notes

Daily

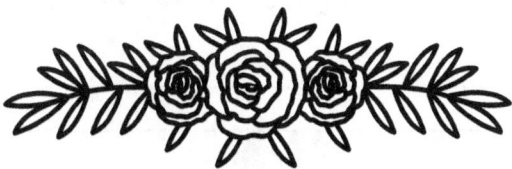

Date
_____

SELF-ESTEEM

Something I did well today

_____

_____

I had fun today when...

_____

_____

I felt proud when...

_____

_____

I had a positive experience with...

_____

_____

Something good I did for someone else

_____

_____

I felt good about myself when...

_____

_____

Today was interesting because...

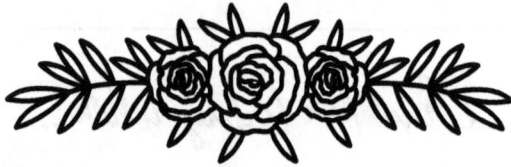

_____

_____

_____

_____

Today's Positive Emotions

Today's Negative Emotions

_____

_____

Weekly
BEHAVIOR TRACKER

Unhealthy Habits

	M	T	W	T	F	S	S
Substance Abuse							
Self-harm							
Over spending							
Over eating							
Lying							
Stealing/Cheating							
Violence/Anger							

What did I struggle most with this week?

How did I deal with my depression and issues this week?

Notes

Daily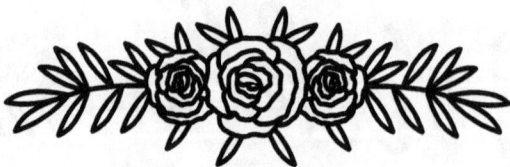

SELF-ESTEEM

Date ____

Something I did well today

_____

_____

I had fun today when...

_____

_____

I felt proud when...

_____

_____

I had a positive experience with...

_____

_____

Something good I did for someone else

_____

_____

I felt good about myself when...

_____

_____

Today was interesting because...

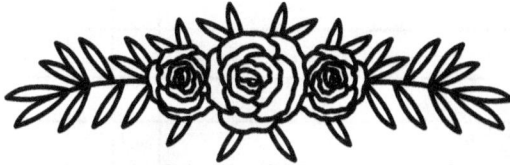

_____

_____

_____

_____

Today's Positive Emotions

Today's Negative Emotions

_____

_____

Weekly
BEHAVIOR TRACKER

Unhealthy Habits

	M	T	W	T	F	S	S
Substance Abuse							
Self-harm							
Over spending							
Over eating							
Lying							
Stealing/Cheating							
Violence/Anger							

What did I struggle most with this week?

How did I deal with my depression and issues this week?

Notes

Daily

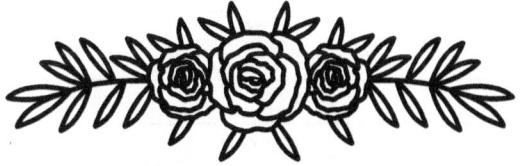

Date
_____

SELF-ESTEEM

Something I did well today

_____

_____

I had fun today when...

_____

_____

I felt proud when...

_____

_____

I had a positive experience with...

_____

_____

Something good I did for someone else

_____

_____

I felt good about myself when...

_____

_____

Today was interesting because...

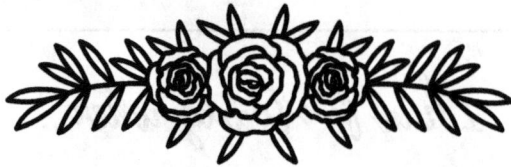

_____

_____

_____

_____

Today's Positive Emotions

Today's Negative Emotions

_____

_____

Weekly
BEHAVIOR TRACKER

Unhealthy Habits

	M	T	W	T	F	S	S
Substance Abuse							
Self-harm							
Over spending							
Over eating							
Lying							
Stealing/Cheating							
Violence/Anger							

What did I struggle most with this week?

How did I deal with my depression and issues this week?

Notes

Daily

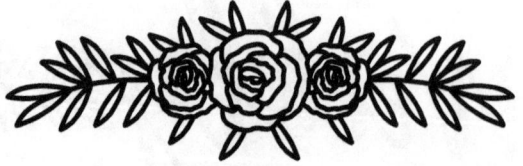

Date

____

SELF-ESTEEM

Something I did well today

_____

_____

I had fun today when...

_____

_____

I felt proud when...

_____

_____

I had a positive experience with...

_____

_____

Something good I did for someone else

_____

_____

I felt good about myself when...

_____

_____

Today was interesting because...

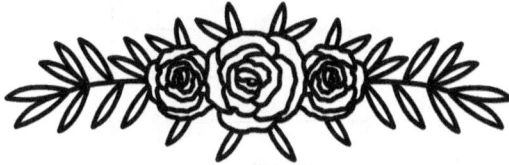

_____

_____

_____

_____

Today's Positive Emotions

Today's Negative Emotions

_____

_____

Weekly
BEHAVIOR TRACKER

Unhealthy Habits

	M	T	W	T	F	S	S
Substance Abuse							
Self-harm							
Over spending							
Over eating							
Lying							
Stealing/Cheating							
Violence/Anger							

What did I struggle most with this week?

How did I deal with my depression and issues this week?

Notes

Daily

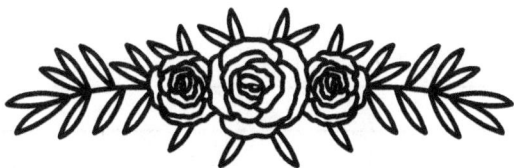

Date ____

SELF-ESTEEM

Something I did well today

_____

_____

I had fun today when...

_____

_____

I felt proud when...

_____

_____

I had a positive experience with...

_____

_____

Something good I did for someone else

_____

_____

I felt good about myself when...

_____

_____

Today was interesting because...

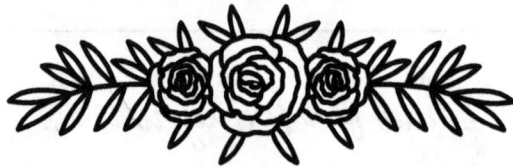

_____

_____

_____

_____

Today's Positive Emotions

Today's Negative Emotions

_____

_____

Weekly
BEHAVIOR TRACKER

Unhealthy Habits

	M	T	W	T	F	S	S
Substance Abuse							
Self-harm							
Over spending							
Over eating							
Lying							
Stealing/Cheating							
Violence/Anger							

What did I struggle most with this week?

How did I deal with my depression and issues this week?

Notes

Daily

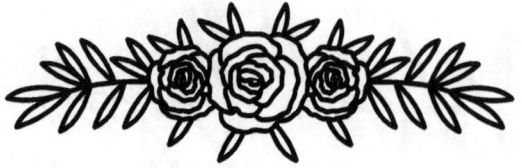

Date _____

SELF-ESTEEM

Something I did well today

_____

_____

I had fun today when...

_____

_____

I felt proud when...

_____

_____

I had a positive experience with...

_____

_____

Something good I did for someone else

_____

_____

I felt good about myself when...

_____

_____

Today was interesting because...

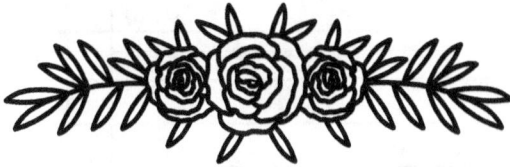

_____

_____

_____

_____

Today's Positive Emotions

Today's Negative Emotions

_____

_____

Weekly
BEHAVIOR TRACKER

Unhealthy Habits

	M	T	W	T	F	S	S
Substance Abuse							
Self-harm							
Over spending							
Over eating							
Lying							
Stealing/Cheating							
Violence/Anger							

What did I struggle most with this week?

How did I deal with my depression and issues this week?

Notes

Daily

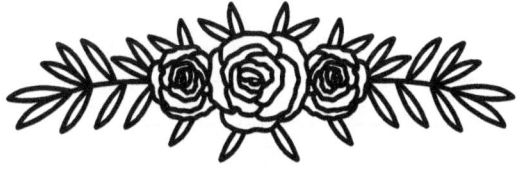

SELF-ESTEEM

Date _____

Something I did well today

_____

_____

I had fun today when...

_____

_____

I felt proud when...

_____

_____

I had a positive experience with...

_____

_____

Something good I did for someone else

_____

_____

I felt good about myself when...

_____

_____

Today was interesting because...

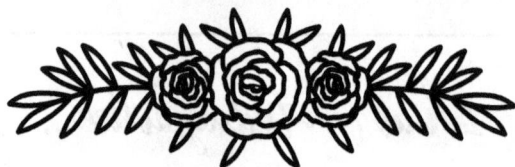

_____

_____

_____

_____

Today's Positive Emotions

Today's Negative Emotions

_____

_____

Weekly
BEHAVIOR TRACKER

Unhealthy Habits

	M	T	W	T	F	S	S
Substance Abuse							
Self-harm							
Over spending							
Over eating							
Lying							
Stealing/Cheating							
Violence/Anger							

What did I struggle most with this week?

How did I deal with my depression and issues this week?

Notes

Daily

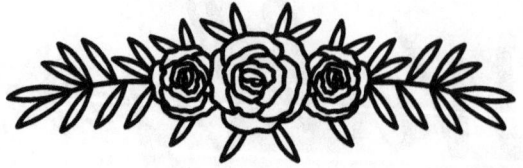

Date
_____ SELF-ESTEEM

Something I did well today

_____
_____

I had fun today when...

_____
_____

I felt proud when...

_____
_____

I had a positive experience with...

_____
_____

Something good I did for someone else

_____
_____

I felt good about myself when...

_____

_____

Today was interesting because...

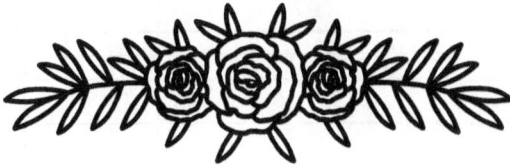

_____

_____

_____

_____

Today's Positive Emotions

Today's Negative Emotions

_____

_____

Weekly
BEHAVIOR TRACKER

Unhealthy Habits

	M	T	W	T	F	S	S
Substance Abuse							
Self-harm							
Over spending							
Over eating							
Lying							
Stealing/Cheating							
Violence/Anger							

What did I struggle most with this week?

How did I deal with my depression and issues this week?

Notes

Daily

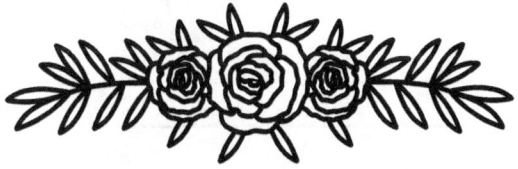

Date
____

SELF-ESTEEM

Something I did well today

_____

_____

I had fun today when...

_____

_____

I felt proud when...

_____

_____

I had a positive experience with...

_____

_____

Something good I did for someone else

_____

_____

I felt good about myself when...

_____

_____

Today was interesting because...

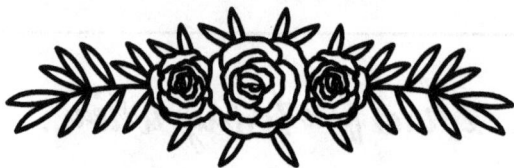

_____

_____

_____

_____

Today's Positive Emotions

Today's Negative Emotions

_____

_____

Weekly
BEHAVIOR TRACKER

Unhealthy Habits

	M	T	W	T	F	S	S
Substance Abuse							
Self-harm							
Over spending							
Over eating							
Lying							
Stealing/Cheating							
Violence/Anger							

What did I struggle most with this week?

How did I deal with my depression and issues this week?

Notes

Daily
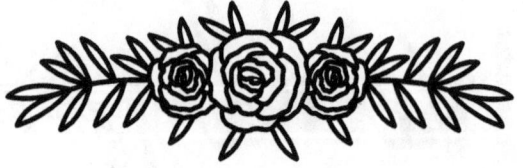

Date
____

SELF-ESTEEM

Something I did well today

_____
_____

I had fun today when...

_____
_____

I felt proud when...

_____
_____

I had a positive experience with...

_____
_____

Something good I did for someone else

_____
_____

I felt good about myself when...

_____
_____

Today was interesting because...

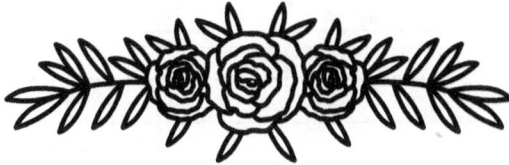

_____
_____
_____
_____

Today's Positive Emotions

Today's Negative Emotions

_____
_____

Weekly
BEHAVIOR TRACKER

Unhealthy Habits

	M	T	W	T	F	S	S
Substance Abuse							
Self-harm							
Over spending							
Over eating							
Lying							
Stealing/Cheating							
Violence/Anger							

What did I struggle most with this week?

How did I deal with my depression and issues this week?

Notes

Daily

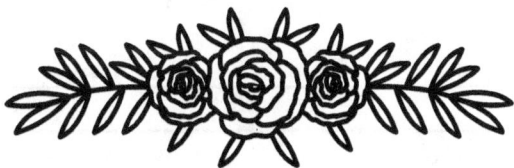

Date
_____

SELF-ESTEEM

Something I did well today

_____

_____

I had fun today when...

_____

_____

I felt proud when...

_____

_____

I had a positive experience with...

_____

_____

Something good I did for someone else

_____

_____

I felt good about myself when...

_____

_____

Today was interesting because...

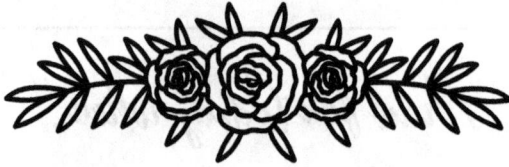

_____

_____

_____

_____

Today's Positive Emotions

Today's Negative Emotions

_____

_____

Weekly
BEHAVIOR TRACKER

Unhealthy Habits

	M	T	W	T	F	S	S
Substance Abuse							
Self-harm							
Over spending							
Over eating							
Lying							
Stealing/Cheating							
Violence/Anger							

What did I struggle most with this week?

How did I deal with my depression and issues this week?

Notes

Daily

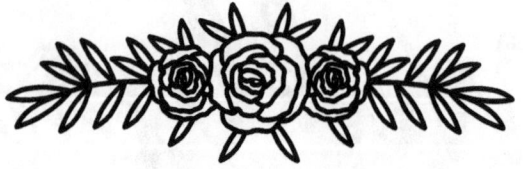

Date

____

SELF-ESTEEM

Something I did well today

_____
_____

I had fun today when...

_____
_____

I felt proud when...

_____
_____

I had a positive experience with...

_____
_____

Something good I did for someone else

_____
_____

I felt good about myself when...

_____

_____

Today was interesting because...

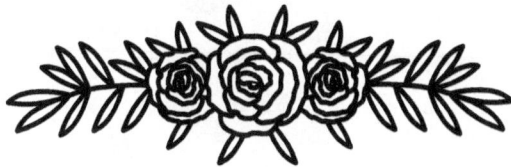

_____

_____

_____

_____

Today's Positive Emotions

Today's Negative Emotions

_____

_____

www.ingramcontent.com/pod-product-compliance
Lightning Source LLC
Chambersburg PA
CBHW051035030426
42336CB00015B/2890